Juicing for cancer recipes:

A detailed recipe book for cancer

By

Crystal M. Thompson

DISCLAIMER PAGE

Table of Content

CHAPTER 1

For a long time, juice for cancer has been a popular alternative to cancer therapy. You are not alone if you want to cure your issues organically. Many individuals employ alternative, natural cancer treatments.

A typical method is to include a healthy diet so that your body has all it needs to fight back and protect itself in order to recover. What is an excellent method to get a lot of nutrients into your body? Juicing, that's right! Juice for cancer is an excellent approach for cancer patients to get critical vitamins and minerals.

For numerous legal reasons, I cannot and will not say that juicing for cancer would cure it.

I can state, however, that I have had several testimonies from my loyal site visitors stating that it worked for them. I can also state that I know juice and healthy nourishment help the body perform amazing things!

Even if you are having chemotherapy or radiation, I am certain that a healthy diet and a daily "juice for cancer" may help your body get through.

Juices should be drunk as soon as possible after processing. This is due to the fact that they oxidize fast. If you can't drink it right away, freeze it (ideally in a glass jar with a cover). Otherwise, you may add an anti-oxidant to the mixture, such as lemon juice, to halt the oxidation process.

To understand why cancer and juicing are the topics of this week's post,

I believe it is necessary to first refresh our memory on some of the fundamentals of cancer.

Cancer includes some very aberrant cell processes. A cancer cell, which was formerly a normal healthy cell in the body, suddenly fails to function or mature normally. The cell's DNA alters its regular function by turning on or off genes that safeguard the cell.

Following that, the cell does not age and die as normal cells are designed to do (apoptosis) but instead creates an increasing number of these reprogrammed cells. They become heavy feeders on your energy and severely deplete your body's energy resources since they grow and multiply so quickly.

If left untreated, these aberrant cancer cells multiply to become malignant tumors, which subsequently move to other regions of the body (metastasize).

Cancer cells, as previously said, are voracious consumers of your energy stores.

If you have cancer, you will have noticed that you are significantly more exhausted than you were before. If you eat a typical American diet, you will undoubtedly be deficient in critical nutrients that might otherwise help your body fight cancer cells more effectively.

The fact is that a robust and healthy immune system, as well as the preservation of our genes, are critical in this struggle, and this necessitates a lot more "supplies" such as vitamins, minerals, antioxidants, and other nutrients.

The National Cancer Institute's "5-A-Day For Better Health" campaign, which was launched in 1991, promotes 5 to 9 servings of fruits and vegetables each day to impact improved health outcomes. However, a significant number of Americans fail to meet these targets.

Many cancer patients find it difficult to consume enough fruits and vegetables to truly affect their health in a good manner, leaving their bodies starved for crucial nutrients at the cellular level.

For many years, cancer patients have used fresh, raw juicing. Some cancer sufferers report that juicing helped them survive their disease when no other therapy was available.

Some people utilized fresh raw juices alone, while others drank 2 or 3 drinks per day to augment an already healthy diet, providing fuel to their cancer-fighting capacities. These examples may be found in a variety of publications as well as on the internet.

The greatest juice variety comes from nature's own containers: fresh fruits and vegetables. Fresh juice is high in phytochemicals and vitamins that combat cancer and are readily absorbed by the body.

Did you know that? 1 cup of carrot or celery juice contains the majority of the nutrients present in 5 cups of those veggies chopped up.

A juice extractor is required to begin juicing.

For individuals who don't have one but want to purchase one, department shops sell a variety of models ranging from $20 to $300.

If you juice often, high-tech features (such as the capacity to process entire, uncut fruits) are worth the additional money. Otherwise, a simple model will suffice.

Citrus juicers and juice extractors are the two sorts.

Extractors are more adaptable; most contain a pulp collector that extracts the fiber (which is why you should still eat full fruits and veggies).

Look for a machine with dishwasher-safe or easily-cleanable components.

Read over the instructions that come with your juicer to get acquainted with how it operates as well as the recipes offered. After each usage, properly clean your juicer with hot soapy water.

PLEASE NOTE: These dishes are NOT suitable for individuals following the Low Microbial Diet (LMD).

Ingredients:
Apple Juice - Carrot Juice
Three to four medium carrots

1 Granny Smith apple, medium

Carrot juice is pleasantly sweet and complements the sharpness of the apples. When purchasing Granny Smiths, pick firm ones for a clearer juice.

10 ounces equals 200 calories, 0g fat, 49g carbohydrates, 4g protein.

Cucumber, celery, and spinach juice
2 cups (4 oz) packed spinach

1 cup cucumber

1 celery sprig

Because the celery isn't overbearing, the spinach and cucumber juices can shine. Spinach is high in calcium, iron, and potassium.

10 ounces contains 139 calories, 1 gram of fat, 35 grams of carbohydrates, and 1 gram of protein.

Juice of pineapple, blueberry, and ginger
14 pineapples

1 cup fresh blueberries

14-12 inch slice of fresh ginger

Blueberries are high in antioxidants, which have been found to help prevent cancer. When mixed with pineapple, ginger improves digestion and creates a South Pacific atmosphere.

12 ounces equals 80 calories, 0 grams of fat, 16 grams of carbohydrates, and 7 grams of protein.

I'm not here to advocate juicing as a cancer cure, but it is indisputable that for many people, it may play a significant part in their recovery process. This is a personal decision for you, and we want to give you some information (by no means all of the information available) to assist you in making the best option for you.

CHAPTER 2

So, let's look at some of the benefits and drawbacks of juicing while you have cancer.

Benefits of Juicing
- Fresh raw juices will revitalize you while offering concentrated amounts of strong anti-cancer, anti-tumor, and anti-inflammatory vitamins, minerals, enzymes, phytochemicals, and antioxidants that the body can readily absorb. Citrus juice includes around 60 flavonoids and 170 phytochemicals, which is equivalent to "calling in the troops" to battle inflammation and cancer.

- **Immune system support** - A healthy immune system is critical in the battle against cancer. Cancer, as well as chemotherapy and radiation, damage the immune system. We need a robust immune system to identify and eliminate aberrant cancer cells. Cancer patients, in particular, must include extra immune-boosting techniques in their diet to combat the spread of malignant cells.

- **Easier to absorb and digest** - Many cancer patients find it difficult to eat a full meal of prepared vegetables, much alone raw vegetables. Fresh raw juices keep all the goodness alive, such as vitamins and antioxidants, as opposed to boiling the vegetables, which typically lose the nutrient content.

Juices may be simpler for some cancer patients to eat, particularly if they have difficulty chewing, or swallowing, have a weak appetite, or experiencing recurrent nausea.When you drink fresh raw juices, you get highly concentrated vitamins, minerals, and enzymes, among other things, that quickly enter the circulation, absorbing all of the nutritional advantages, giving you more energy, and allowing part of your digestive organs to rest.

- Fresh raw juices are capable of boosting the activity of the intestines, liver, bile, and kidneys, which has the effect of promoting the breakdown and removal of harmful substances and waste products from the body due to their high water content.

The Downside of Juicing
- **Lacks Healthy Fiber - Many juicers create a lot of pulp, which is frequently discarded. This pulp includes fiber from the skins and peels of the juiced whole vegetables, as well as part of the goodness. Because the fiber content has been eliminated, juicing alone may cause unwanted digestive difficulties. Many cancer patients suffer from digestive difficulties such as constipation or diarrhea, and fiber is an important component in promoting good bowel habits. If you are especially ill or unable to eat regularly, you may be able to take your fresh juices with an extra fiber supplement, such as stirring in some Fibertone Powder, to ensure that your body receives the fiber it needs.**

- **Too Much Sugar** - Juicing may lead to excessive sugar intake, particularly in diabetics or those with quickly developing malignancies. It is true that juicing, particularly with fruits, raises blood sugar levels. Aside from that, cancer cells need a lot of sugar to multiply so quickly, and glucose is high on their food list. Fresh juices will include varying levels of simple sugars, such as fructose. However, raw fresh juices do not contain refined sugars.

- **Juicing on its own is not a balanced diet** - Juicing on its own lacks a diverse assortment of protein, complex carbs, and lipids. Protein balances the juice's carbs, while fats aid in the absorption of fat-soluble vitamins and minerals.

These foods should ideally be included in a well-balanced diet that includes juicing.

- When it comes to fresh raw juices, it is advisable to keep them low in sugar if you have cancer or diabetes. Green juices* created from green vegetables and leaves are particularly beneficial since they are often low in sugar and rich in many of the nutrients required to combat cancer. They contain chlorophyll, which helps to filter the blood, create red blood cells, detoxify and repair the body, and deliver quick energy to the body.

CHAPTER 3

Blueberry, Pomegranate, and Red Cabbage
This powerful anti-cancer juice recipe includes freshly squeezed pomegranate, red cabbage, and blueberry juice. Their antioxidant-rich components and anti-inflammatory capabilities combine to provide one of the greatest cancer-killing juices that may be used with other treatment methods.

Red Juice that Fights Cancer
Because cabbage juice has a natural healing impact on our gut lining, red cabbage in particular is even more nutrient-dense owing to its pigmented hue and is an ideal addition for producing an anti-inflammatory juice.

The strong taste of red cabbage is wonderfully countered by the sweet and sour flavors of pomegranate and blueberry, resulting in a gorgeous red and magenta-colored drink.

This fresh juice is an excellent method to increase your intake of cancer-fighting polyphenols and vitamins. The components are readily absorbed by the body in this condition, which is particularly advantageous for persons who have digestive disorders and poor absorption.

You just need three ingredients to prepare this cancer-killing juice:

Pomegranates
Cabbage in red
Blueberries
How to Prepare the Juice
A juicer or a blender may be used to extract the juice.

Because pomegranate seeds (arils) have a bitter flavor when crushed, I found that using a juicer improved the taste. However, both function well.
It is also critical to choose a berry "friendly" juicer, particularly if you use a slow masticating juicer. Blueberries have a soft pulp, and a cheaper one does not extract enough juice. The pulp contains the majority of the juice.

Alternatively, you may squeeze the blueberries with a cheesecloth by hand and add them to the pomegranate and cabbage juice afterward.

Once prepared, drink this anti-cancer juice soon away to avoid nutrient loss. The flavor isn't horrible; in fact, it's very excellent. The only drawback is that the cabbage scent is rather strong, so you may want to cover your nose while drinking it.

How Does This Anti-Cancer Red Juice Work?

Cancer-Preventing Properties of Pomegranate

Pomegranate has been demonstrated to have several medical benefits, including antioxidant and anti-inflammatory effects that aid in the prevention and development of cancer.

Pomegranate extracts preferentially suppress the development of breast cancer, prostate cancer, colon cancer, and lung cancer cells in culture, according to a new study.

Pomegranate has also been demonstrated to improve the efficacy of several chemotherapy medicines while shielding against their negative side effects.

The Functions of Red Cabbage and Blueberries
It is well known that cruciferous vegetables are high in bioactive components, particularly sulfur-containing molecules that have been shown to prevent cancer. The presence of anthocyanins, which have considerable anti-oxidant action, distinguishes red cabbage from other sulfur-containing substances.

Anthocyanins (found in red cabbage and blueberries) have been shown to have anti-carcinogenic and pro-apoptotic (programmed cancer cell death) properties. Furthermore, in vivo studies have indicated that dietary anthocyanins may suppress gastrointestinal malignancies and prevent metastasis.

How to Get the Most Out of Your Diet
Cancer often motivates individuals to
reconsider their food, daily activities,
and lifestyle in order to do their part to
remain healthy. After a cancer diagnosis,
nutritional supplements and juicing are
two simple strategies to keep your body
nourished with the nutrients it needs.
However, there are a few things you
should be aware of before making
dietary changes.

Juicing
Why should individuals with cancer drink
juice?
Juicing may help your body absorb
nutrients from fruits and vegetables,
strengthen your immune system, remove
toxins from your body, promote
digestion, and aid in weight reduction.
Although it has not been established that
juicing is more beneficial than eating
conventional fruits and vegetables,

juicing may bring diversity to your diet as well as make it simpler to absorb the nutrients that you need on a daily basis. Some individuals prefer juicing instead of eating entire fruits and veggies. It is especially beneficial for cancer patients if their perception of taste has altered, they have dry mouth, or they have difficulty swallowing full meals.

Is it possible to juice too much?
If you decide to start juicing, keep in mind that "too much juicing" might be dangerous. Overuse of juicing might cause diarrhea and excessive sugar intake in diabetics. It is, as in everything, It is critical to do this in moderation. Juicing is ideal when combined with a balanced diet in general and should not be used in lieu of expert medical treatment.

What should I do first?
A juicer should be used instead of a blender.
Getting a juicer that maintains the peel and pulp in the juice is healthier since the peel and pulp contain a lot of nutrients.
Fresh juice is superior to store-bought juice.
Try to find food that is free of holes and bruises.
Before juicing, wash the fruits and vegetables.
Drink immediately after juicing; juices will not keep fresh in the refrigerator for more than a few hours.
Which fruits and veggies are the greatest to use?

Apple, pineapple, papaya, berries, orange, cantaloupe, and grapes are the finest fruits for juicing. Choose antioxidant-rich fruits. Carrots, cabbage, broccoli, celery, parsley, kale, spinach, and beets are among the finest vegetables for juicing. Carrots are particularly wonderful for juicing since they give a pleasant flavor, are abundant in nutrients, and have a high beta-carotene content, which aids in cancer prevention. Don't be intimidated by juicing veggies! Juiced veggies may seem weird at first, but with the correct ingredients, they can be surprisingly palatable.

Supplements for Nutrition
If you have or have had cancer, you have most certainly attempted to complement your diet with nutritional supplements. Vitamins, minerals, plants, and amino acids are examples of nutritional and

dietary supplements. Here's some advice on how to include vitamins in your diet.

Benefits
The two primary advantages of
nutritional supplements are:

Immune system booster
Assist in reducing the negative effects of
chemotherapy and radiation treatment.
Because it is difficult for the immune
system to detect cancer cells as
aberrant, they often do not assault them.
While nutritional supplements can not
replace drugs given by physicians, if you
can support your body by boosting your
immune system, you will be able to fight
illness more effectively. It is critical to
keep your doctor informed while utilizing
nutritional supplements.
Consult Your Doctor
It is important to consult with your
doctor before making any dietary
adjustments.

You should acquire all of the information, as well as the kind and quantity of supplements you want to take. This is critical to prevent any supplement adverse effects or hazards associated with taking them with other drugs.

D vitamin
There are conflicting findings when it comes to including vitamin D in your diet, yet it is one of the most investigated vitamins for cancer. Many individuals are vitamin D deficient in general; taking vitamin D is appealing to cancer patients because of its function in cell formation. Vitamin D tablets help compensate for time spent in the sun, which patients with cancer are unable to do much of.

Iron

Fatigue is one of the negative effects of cancer therapy. People feel weariness on a variety of levels, with iron deficiency

and anemia (induced by chemotherapy) playing a significant role. If you take vitamin C with meals, your body may absorb more iron from the diet.

Antioxidants, garlic, green tea
Certain foods may assist in supplementing your diet in ways that are comparable to dietary supplements. Including natural garlic in your diet has the potential to enhance your immune system and may have cancer-fighting properties. Green tea may be able to inhibit the growth of blood vessels in malignancies.
Fruits and vegetables include antioxidants that may aid in the battle against cancer. Vitamins A, C, and E, as well as selenium and some chemicals in

green tea and melatonin, are
antioxidants.

Supplement Misconceptions

Many individuals feel that since
supplements are offered over the
counter, they do not need to be cautious
about what they take. They also feel that
"the more the better"; nevertheless, this
is not the case. Other common
misunderstandings include that if the
container says "all-natural," it is natural,
that just because you've heard of it
before means it's safe, that it won't
conflict with your other drugs, and that
just because it's FDA-approved means
it's safe for you. Be wary of these
common myths.

There are advantages to studying nutritional supplements and adopting dietary modifications, but none of these changes should be done without first seeing your doctor.

Juicing may seem to be a health trend, but there are advantages to juicing for cancer patients.

Begin by experimenting with only a few fruits or veggies for your mixtures.

Then you may experiment with different combinations! Slowly introduce this new dietary approach to avoid shocking your body.
A Beta Carotene Superfood
1/3 cantaloupe, rind included
Three carrots
1 orange (peeled)
Excellent Antioxidant Booster
4 pitted apricots
6 strawberries, big

A Rejuvenating Juice
four big carrots

4 broccoli stems
1 garlic bulb

Juice from a Veggie Medley

6 carrots (medium)
1 beet (with leaves)
three huge tomatoes
2–3 big handfuls spinach
1/8 cabbage head

2 to 3 kale leaves
1 red bell pepper to 1 red bell pepper
1 medium celery stalk
1 tablespoon yellow onion
1 garlic clove
Optional: 1/2 bunch parsley
(If desired, add spices such as chili
powder, turmeric, and so on.)
**Regularity Mix (Warning: This mix
contains a lot of fiber!)**

2 plums
2 slices of tiny apples or pears
1-2 tablespoons powdered flax seeds or
psyllium husk (optional) for added fiber

Try some of these juicing recipes to see
what works best for you! Always
remember to eat in moderation.